To The Reader.

I dedicate this book to all patients and professionals who understand the value of careful and well-guided recovery after surgery.

To my patients, whose trust and commitment to their own health are the motivation to constantly improve my work. To the community of massage therapists and health professionals who dedicate their careers to providing relief, recovery, and quality of life to so many.

This book is the result of my journey and commitment to excellence in post-operative lymphatic drainage, with the hope of bringing clarity and real results to those seeking effective and informed recovery.

With deep respect and professionalism, The Massage Therapist, João Mario Pereira.

Introduction

Manual lymphatic drainage is a therapeutic technique that has become essential in the recovery of patients undergoing plastic surgery. Understanding its importance and the benefits it can bring is fundamental for anyone seeking an effective recovery process. This book is a straightforward guide that seeks to clarify and inform about manual lymphatic drainage, covering everything from its history to its specific applications after surgical procedures.

Table of Contents

Chapter 1

A Little History of Manual Lymphatic Drainage

Manual lymphatic drainage, a technique that is now widely recognized in health and aesthetic treatments, has its roots in antiquity but was officially structured in the 20th century. The lymphatic system, crucial for maintaining immunity and the circulation of bodily fluids, intrigued ancient physicians who, despite limited knowledge, already recognized the importance of keeping the body in balance. However, the lymphatic system remained a mystery for many centuries, being studied more thoroughly only in the Renaissance.

In the 17th century, Danish physician Thomas Bartholin was one of the first to describe the function of lymphatic vessels in detail. He realized that this system was distinct from the blood system, and his discovery opened doors for a clearer understanding of the role of lymph in the body's defense. Even with these advances, it was only in the early 20th century that manual lymphatic drainage began to take shape as a therapeutic technique. In the 1930s, Danish therapists Emil and Estrid Vodder developed the method that is now known as Manual Lymphatic Drainage (MLD).

Emil Vodder noticed that many patients who presented with colds and chronic diseases had swollen lymph nodes. He began to apply gentle and specific touches to these regions, which resulted in the improvement of symptoms. The technique was initially discredited by the scientific community, but over time, its effectiveness was proven by clinical studies and practical observations. MLD began to be recognized as an important tool not only in the relief of lymphatic conditions but also as a complement in post-operative and aesthetic treatments.

The success of manual lymphatic drainage is due to its ability to stimulate the lymphatic system, promoting the removal of toxins, reducing swelling (edema), and accelerating healing, especially after plastic surgery. Over the decades, the technique has evolved, being adapted to different medical and aesthetic needs. Today, it is widely used by physical therapists, aestheticians, and other health professionals worldwide.

Therefore, manual lymphatic drainage is not just a technique but the result of centuries of study and the evolution of knowledge about the human body. In the next chapter, we will explore in more detail how the lymphatic system works and its importance in post-surgical recovery, especially in aesthetic procedures.

Chapter 2

What is Manual Lymphatic Drainage?

Lymphatic drainage is a therapeutic massage technique whose main objective is to stimulate the lymphatic system. This system is fundamental to the body's health, as it works to remove accumulated fluids, toxins, and waste, in addition to playing an essential role in the immune response. Lymphatic drainage is recognized for its positive effects on physical health and general well-being, being used in various situations, from the treatment of clinical conditions to aiding in beauty and aesthetic procedures. Before we delve into lymphatic drainage, it's important to understand how the lymphatic system works.

The lymphatic system is a complex network of vessels, nodes, and organs that permeate the entire body. Among its main functions are:

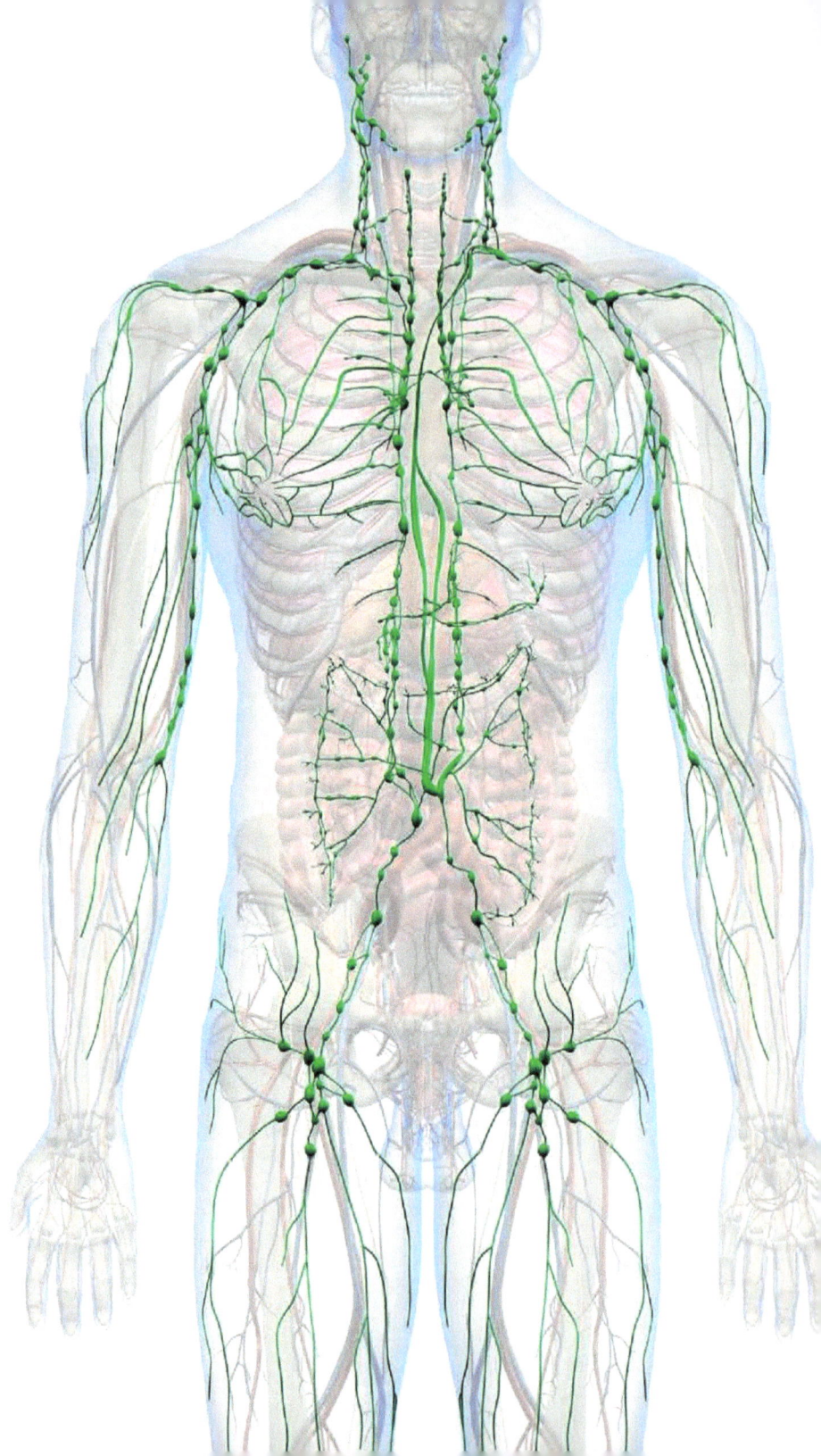

- **Lymph transport:** Lymph is a clear fluid that contains white blood cells, proteins, and cellular debris. Lymphatic vessels transport lymph from tissues to the bloodstream.

- **Cellulite:** Contributes to the reduction of cellulite by stimulating circulation and the elimination of toxins.

- **Stress and Anxiety:** Gentle movements promote relaxation, helping to reduce stress levels.

- **Waste filtration:** Lymph nodes act as filters, removing pathogens and damaged cells from the lymph before it returns to circulation.

- **Immune system activation:** The lymphatic system produces and transports immune cells that help fight infections and diseases.

How Does Lymphatic Drainage Work?

Manual lymphatic drainage is performed through gentle, rhythmic, and directed movements that follow the natural path of the lymphatic vessels. These movements have a direct effect on the flow of lymph, facilitating its circulation and promoting the elimination of toxins from the body. The main aspects of the technique include:

- **Gentle movements:** The pressure used during the massage should be light and gentle, avoiding any discomfort to the patient. The idea is to stimulate the lymph without causing trauma to the tissues.

- **Rhythmic pace:** The cadence of the movements is fundamental. The therapist must maintain a constant rhythm that helps to relax the patient and stimulate drainage.

- **Proper direction:** The movements must be performed in the direction of the lymph nodes, respecting the natural flow of the lymph. This helps to maximize the benefits of drainage.

Benefits of Lymphatic Drainage

Lymphatic drainage offers a range of benefits, both physical and psychological. Some of the main ones include:

- **Reduction of edema:** Helps to reduce swelling caused by fluid retention, being especially effective after surgeries and injuries.

- **Improved blood circulation:** Stimulation of the lymphatic system can also contribute to better blood circulation, promoting tissue oxygenation.

- **Strengthening of the immune system:** By facilitating the removal of toxins and the activation of immune cells, lymphatic drainage can reinforce the body's defense capacity.

- **Relief of stress and anxiety:** The gentle and relaxing movements promote a state of tranquility, helping to reduce stress and anxiety levels.

- **Support in aesthetic treatments:** It is a valued technique in aesthetics, being widely used to improve skin appearance, reduce cellulite, and aid in recovery after aesthetic procedures.

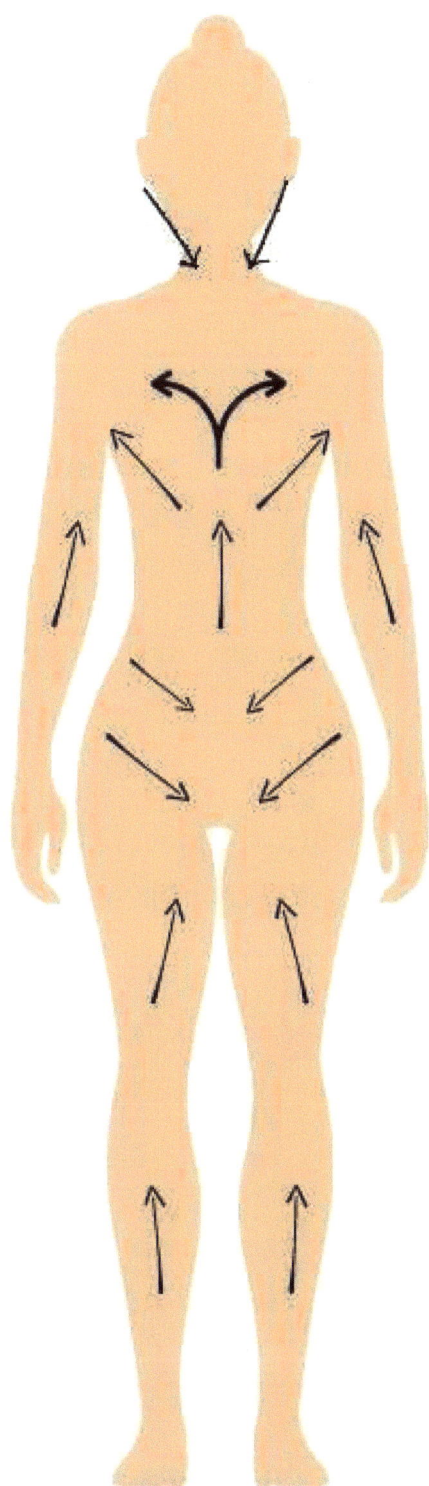

Indications for Lymphatic Drainage

Lymphatic drainage is indicated for various conditions, including:

- **Post-surgery:** It is essential in the recovery of patients who have undergone plastic surgery, helping to reduce swelling and improve healing.

- **Lymphedema:** It is indispensable for patients with chronic fluid retention and lymphatic problems.

- **Cellulite:** It can be used to improve the appearance of cellulite by promoting circulation and the elimination of toxins.

- **Stress conditions:** Individuals who suffer from stress or accumulated tension can benefit from the relaxing effects of MLD.

Conclusion

Lymphatic drainage is a valuable technique that not only improves physical health but also contributes to general well-being. By stimulating the lymphatic system and promoting the elimination of toxins, this technique helps the body to function more efficiently. In a world where health and aesthetics are increasingly interconnected, lymphatic drainage stands out as a powerful tool for those seeking effective recovery and a healthy lifestyle. In the next chapter, we will explore in more depth how the lymphatic system operates and its importance to the health of the organism.

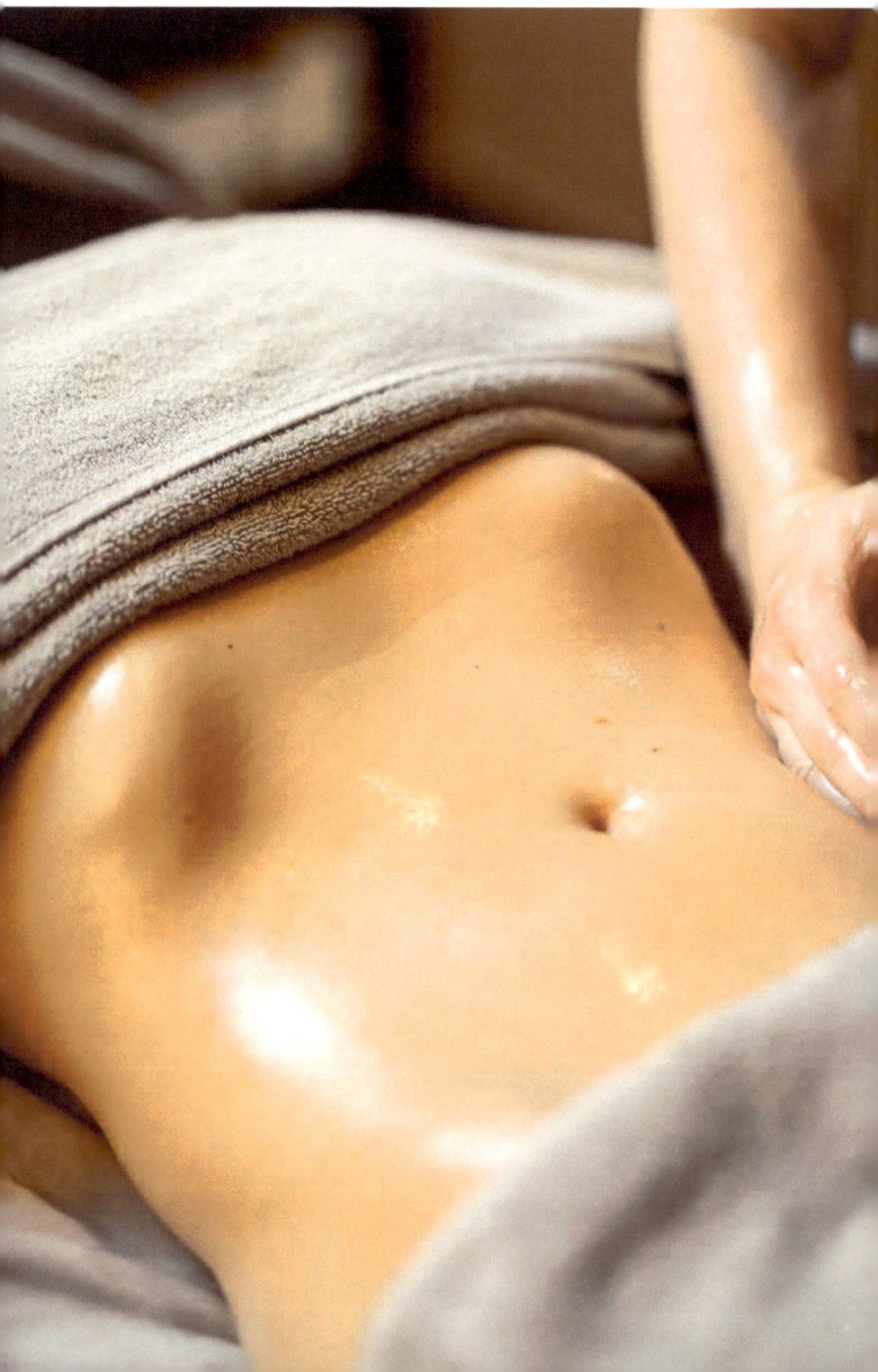

Chapter 3

How the Lymphatic System Works

The lymphatic system is a complex and interconnected network of vessels, nodes, and organs that plays a vital role in immunity and fluid regulation in the body. Understanding its function is essential for applying lymphatic drainage effectively, as this technique depends on the proper functioning of this system to maximize its benefits.

Structure of the Lymphatic System

- **Lymphatic vessels:** Just as veins carry blood, lymphatic vessels carry lymph. They branch throughout the body, forming a network that drains fluids from tissues and transports them back to the bloodstream.

- **Lymph nodes:** Located at strategic points in the body, lymph nodes are small, bean-shaped structures that act as filters for lymph. They contain immune cells that help detect and fight infections and other threats.

14

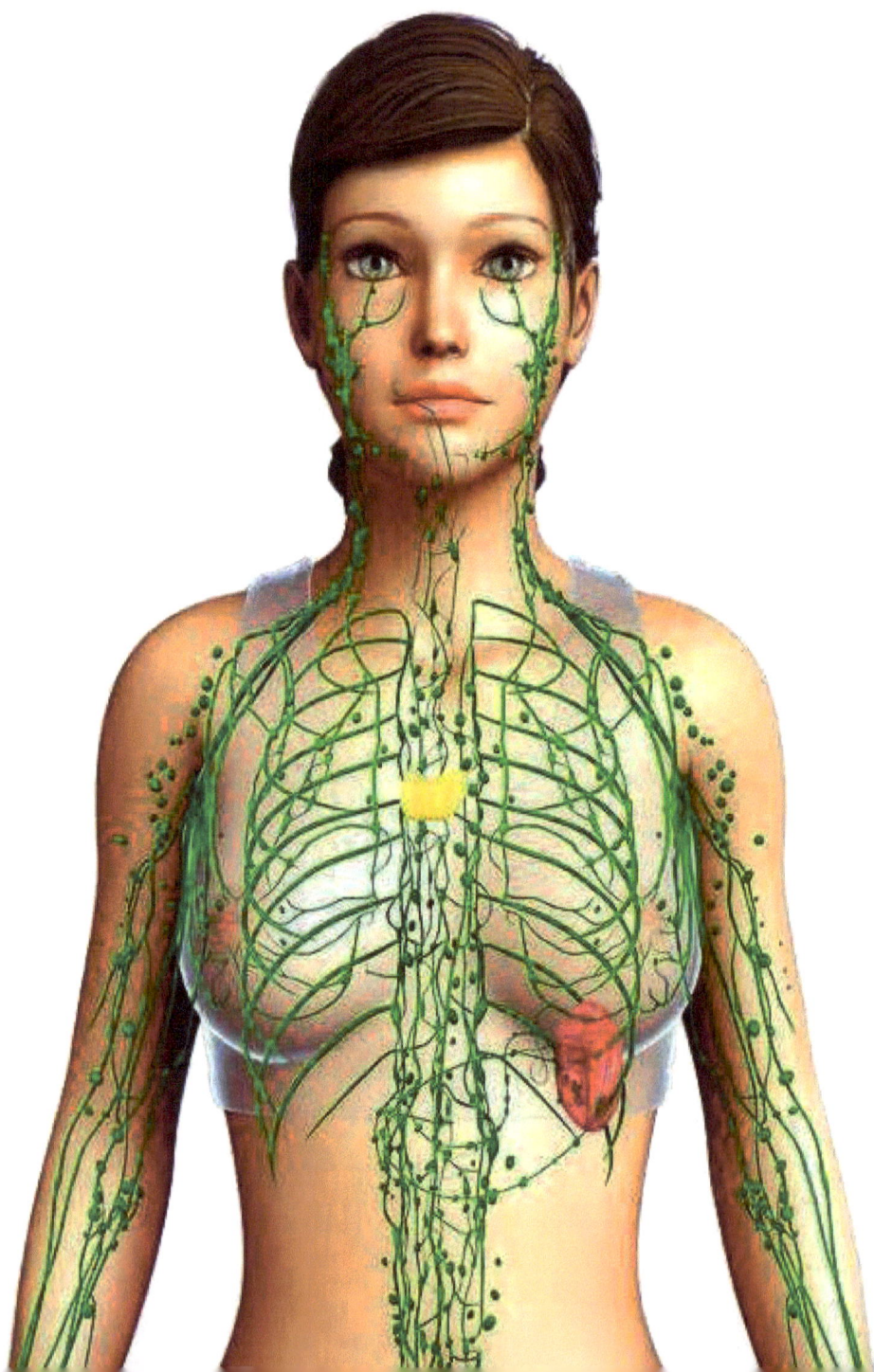

- **Lymphatic organs:** In addition to the nodes, the lymphatic system includes organs such as the spleen and tonsils, which play important roles in the production and storage of immune cells.

Functions of the Lymphatic System

The lymphatic system has several crucial functions for the health of the organism:

- **Immunity:** Lymph nodes filter lymph and capture pathogens, such as bacteria and viruses. The immune cells present in the nodes activate an immune response, helping to protect the body against infections.

- **Fluid regulation:** The lymphatic system plays an important role in regulating the volume of fluids in the body. It collects excess interstitial fluid from tissues and returns it to the bloodstream, helping to prevent swelling.

- **Lipid transport:** After digestion, the lymphatic system transports lipids and fat-soluble vitamins from the intestines to the bloodstream. This process is vital for the absorption of essential nutrients.

Lymph Circulation

Lymph circulation occurs unidirectionally, meaning lymph flows from peripheral areas of the body toward the heart. This process is driven by:

- **Muscle contractions:** The movement of muscles during physical activity presses on the lymphatic vessels, helping to push the lymph forward.
- **Respiratory movements:** The negative pressure created during breathing also aids in the movement of lymph.
- **Lymphatic valves:** the Lymphatic vessels have valves that prevent the backflow of lymph, ensuring that it flows in only one direction.

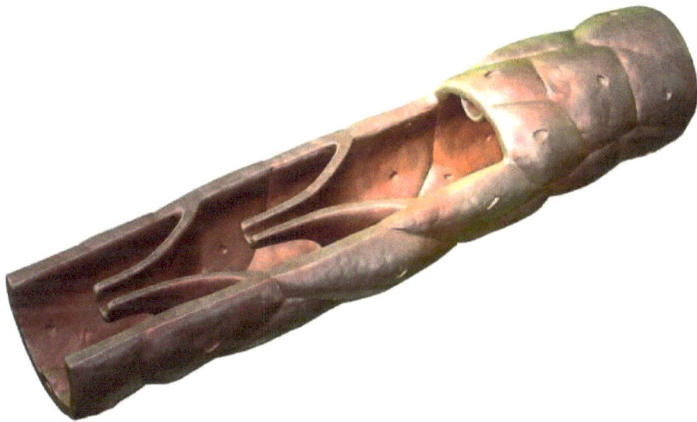

- **Interaction with the Circulatory System:** The lymphatic system is closely interconnected with the circulatory system. Lymph is ultimately drained into the venous system, where it mixes with blood. This interaction is crucial for maintaining fluid balance and proper immune function.

Importance of Lymphatic Drainage

Understanding how the lymphatic system works is fundamental to applying manual lymphatic drainage effectively. The technique takes advantage of the natural functioning of the system, helping to:

- **Increase lymphatic flow:** Gentle and directed movements stimulate the lymphatic vessels, promoting a more efficient flow of lymph.

- **Unblock lymph nodes:** MLD can help release accumulated lymph in the nodes, facilitating filtration and the activation of immune cells.

- **Reduce edema**: By promoting the removal of excess fluids from tissues, lymphatic drainage helps reduce swelling and pressure on the lymphatic vessels.

Conclusion

The lymphatic system plays a fundamental role in maintaining health, acting in immunity and the regulation of body fluids. Understanding its functioning is essential for the effective application of manual lymphatic drainage, a technique that can enhance the benefits of this system. As we continue our journey through the knowledge of lymphatic drainage, in the next chapter, we will explore the benefits and indications of this technique for health and well-being.

Chapter 4

Benefits of Manual Lymphatic Drainage

Manual lymphatic drainage (MLD) is a technique recognized for its various health and wellness benefits. Understanding these benefits is essential, especially for those recovering from plastic surgery or dealing with conditions that affect the lymphatic system. In this chapter, we will explore how MLD can be a valuable tool to improve quality of life and facilitate recovery.

1. **Reduction of swelling:** One of the most notable benefits of manual lymphatic drainage is its ability to reduce swelling, or edema. After surgeries, injuries, or in conditions such as lymphedema, lymph can accumulate in the tissues, causing swelling. MLD helps stimulate lymph flow, facilitating the removal of excess fluids and promoting detoxification.

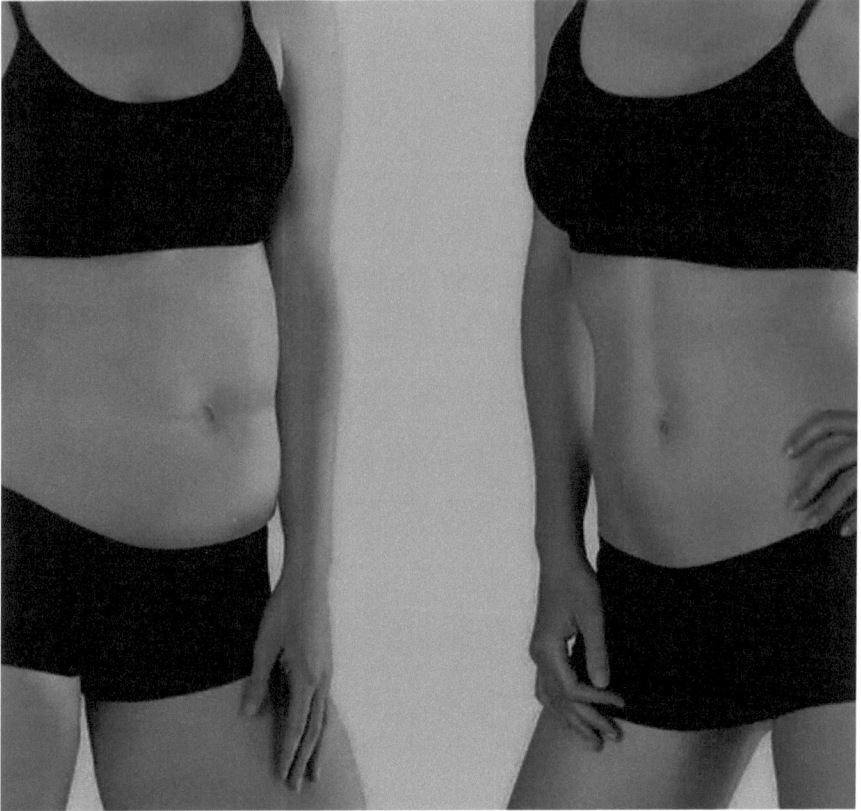

Before   **After**

This effect is particularly important in the post-operative period of plastic surgeries, where fluid retention is common.

2. **Pain relief:** MLD can also provide pain relief. The gentle and rhythmic movements of the technique help relax muscles and release tension, which can result in a decrease in pain

and discomfort. Furthermore, by reducing swelling and improving circulation, lymphatic drainage can contribute to a general sense of well-being, helping patients recover more quickly.

3. **Improved blood circulation:** Manual lymphatic drainage not only stimulates the lymphatic system but also improves blood circulation. By facilitating the flow of lymph, MLD aids in the oxygenation of tissues and the removal of metabolic waste. This improvement in circulation is crucial for recovery, as it ensures that tissues receive the nutrients and oxygen necessary for healing and regeneration.

4. **Relaxation and well-being:** The benefits of MLD go beyond the physical; the technique promotes a deep state of relaxation. The gentle and rhythmic movements help reduce stress and anxiety levels, providing a sense of calm and tranquility. The relaxation generated by MLD not only improves the recovery experience but can also have a

positive impact on the patient's mental and emotional health.

5. **Support for the immune system:** Manual lymphatic drainage plays an important role in activating the immune system. By stimulating the lymph nodes and increasing lymph flow, MLD helps improve the body's ability to fight infections. This is particularly beneficial for patients recovering from surgery, as they may be more susceptible to infections during the recovery period.

6. **Improved skin appearance:** MLD is also a valued technique in aesthetics, as it contributes to improving skin appearance. Through stimulation of circulation and removal of toxins, lymphatic drainage can help tone the skin, reduce cellulite, and promote a healthy glow. These aesthetic benefits are often sought after by those who have undergone plastic surgery or aesthetic procedures, as they help enhance the results.

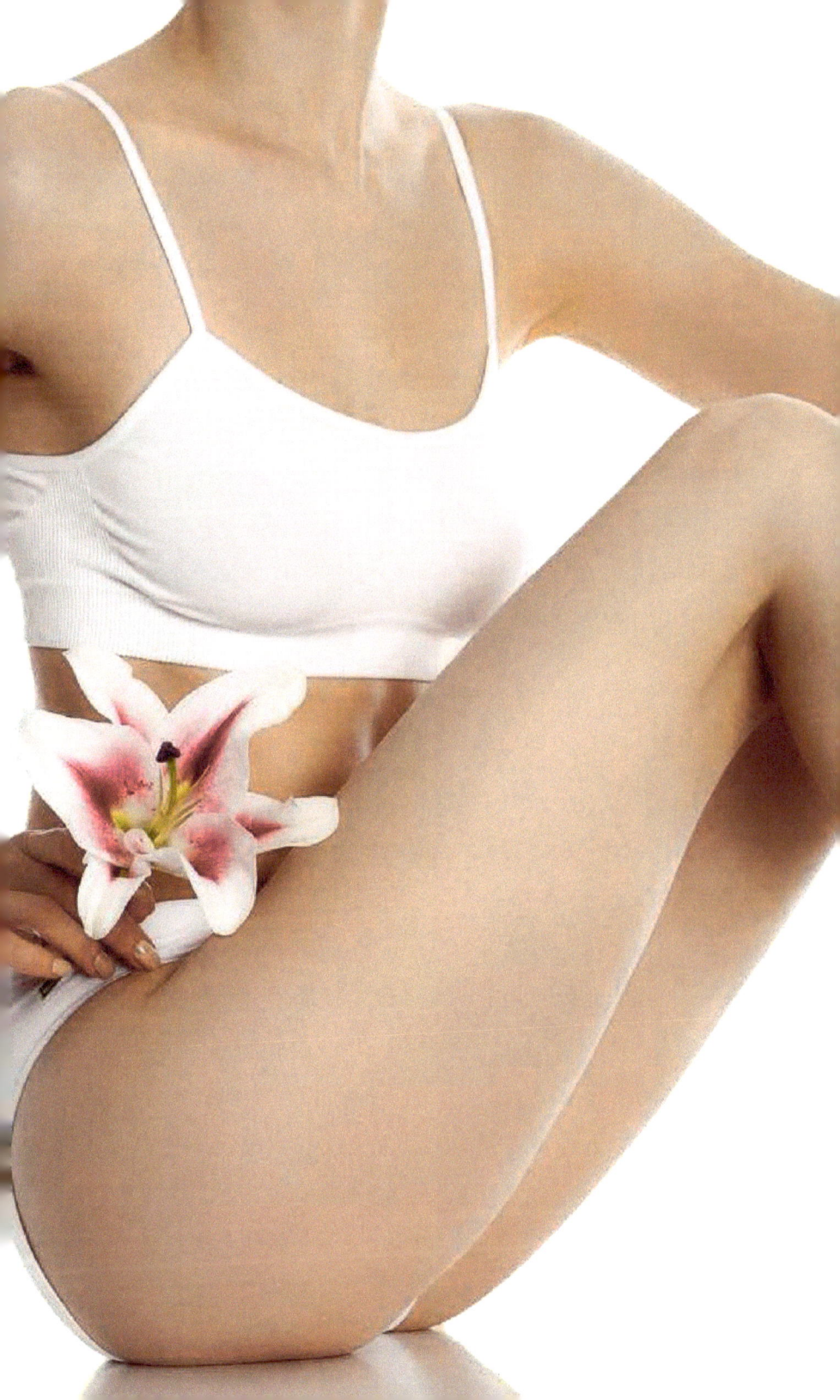

Post-Surgical Indications

After plastic surgeries, manual lymphatic drainage is highly recommended as part of the recovery plan. The technique helps accelerate the healing process by reducing swelling and improving circulation, which is essential for recovery from surgeries such as abdominoplasty, liposuction, and breast augmentation. Patients undergoing these surgeries can benefit significantly from MLD, making it a common practice in aesthetic and rehabilitation clinics.

Conclusion

Manual lymphatic drainage offers a range of benefits that go far beyond simple swelling relief. From promoting blood circulation to strengthening the immune system and improving emotional well-being, MLD is a valuable tool for those seeking to accelerate recovery and improve quality of life. By considering lymphatic drainage as part of the recovery process, especially after plastic surgery, it is possible to maximize results and promote a smoother, more effective recovery. In the next chapter, we will address the specific indications for lymphatic drainage, detailing when and how this technique can be used.

Chapter 5

Importance of Lymphatic Drainage in Post-Operative Care

After plastic surgery, the body undergoes a series of changes and requires special care to ensure proper recovery. One of the most effective methods to aid in this process is manual lymphatic drainage (MLD). This technique not only promotes physical health but also helps in the aesthetic and emotional recovery of patients. In this chapter, we will explore the importance of lymphatic drainage in post-operative care, highlighting its benefits and contributions to a faster and more effective recovery.

1. **Prevention of complications:** After plastic surgery, the body can face various complications, including the accumulation of fluids, which can lead to hematomas and infections. Manual lymphatic drainage acts as a preventive measure, helping to avoid the formation of seromas (accumulation of fluid in cavities) and other problems related to fluid retention.

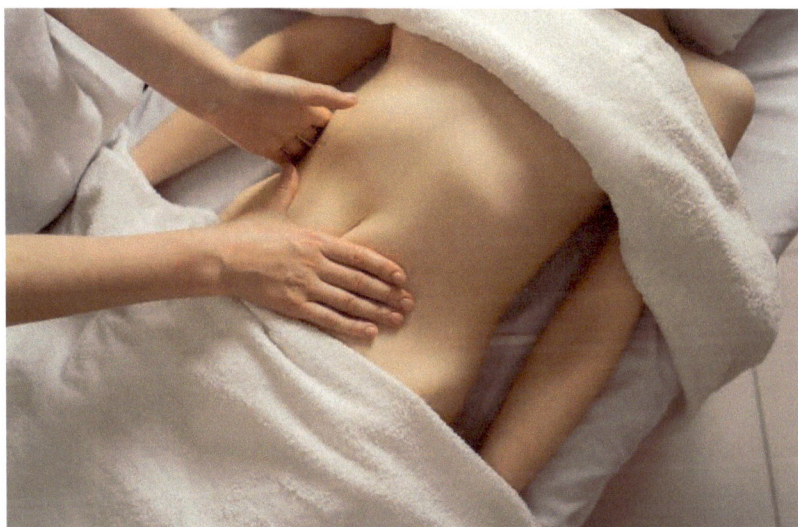

Manual Lymphatic Drainage

By stimulating the flow of lymph and facilitating the drainage of excess fluids, MLD contributes to a smoother and complication-free recovery.

2. **Reduction of swelling:** One of the most common side effects after plastic surgery is swelling. Edema can be uncomfortable and affect the patient's mobility. Manual lymphatic drainage is especially effective in reducing this swelling, as it promotes the removal of excess fluids accumulated in the tissues. With the reduction of edema, patients can experience relief from pressure

and discomfort, making the recovery process more comfortable.

3. **Improved blood circulation:** MLD not only stimulates the lymphatic system but also improves blood circulation. After surgery, it is vital to ensure that tissues receive adequate oxygen and nutrients for healing. The technique facilitates blood flow, promoting better tissue oxygenation and accelerating healing. This is particularly important for areas that may be compromised due to surgical trauma.

4. **Accelerated recovery:** With the combination of complication prevention, swelling reduction, and improved circulation, manual lymphatic drainage significantly contributes to faster recovery. Patients who receive MLD after plastic surgery generally report less discomfort and more efficient recovery. This positive effect can shorten downtime and allow patients to return to their daily activities more quickly.

5. **Improved scar appearance:** Another important aspect of lymphatic drainage in post-operative care is its ability to improve the appearance of scars. MLD helps smooth the tissues around the scar and promotes cell regeneration. With increased circulation and reduced swelling, scars can become less visible, resulting in a more aesthetic and harmonious appearance. This is particularly valuable for patients undergoing procedures that leave scars, such as abdominoplasty and facelifts.

6. **Emotional support:** In addition to physical benefits, manual lymphatic drainage can offer emotional support to recovering patients. The recovery process after plastic surgery can be challenging, and many patients may experience anxiety or stress. MLD, with its gentle and relaxing movements, helps promote a state of calm and tranquility. This can be especially beneficial during the first few post-operative days, when patients may feel vulnerable and concerned about the results.

7. **Indications and Start Times:** It is important to note that manual lymphatic drainage should be started after authorization from the responsible physician, usually a few days after surgery. The timing and frequency of MLD sessions may vary depending on the type of surgery and the individual condition of each patient. Generally, it is recommended to start MLD sessions between 48 to 72 hours after the surgical procedure, continuing for a period that can range from one to several weeks.

Conclusion

Manual lymphatic drainage plays a crucial role in post-operative recovery, offering a range of benefits from preventing complications to improving scar appearance. With its ability to reduce swelling, improve circulation, and provide emotional relief, MLD is a valuable tool for those who have undergone plastic surgery. By including this technique in the recovery plan, patients can enjoy a smoother and more effective experience, contributing to better aesthetic results and a more complete recovery. In the next chapter, we will address the specific indications and contraindications of manual lymphatic drainage, so that readers can better understand when and how this technique can be used.

Chapter 6

When to Start Lymphatic Drainage After Plastic Surgery

Manual lymphatic drainage (MLD) is a highly beneficial technique for post-surgical recovery, especially after aesthetic procedures. However, knowing exactly when to start MLD sessions is crucial to maximize their benefits and ensure patient safety. In this chapter, we will address the guidelines for starting lymphatic drainage, the importance of professional guidance, and how the type of surgery can influence the schedule.

1. **Ideal time to start MLD:** In general, it is recommended to start manual lymphatic drainage around 48 to 72 hours after surgery. This time frame is crucial as it allows the body to begin the initial healing process. During the first few days, swelling and discomfort are more intense, and MLD can help mitigate these symptoms.

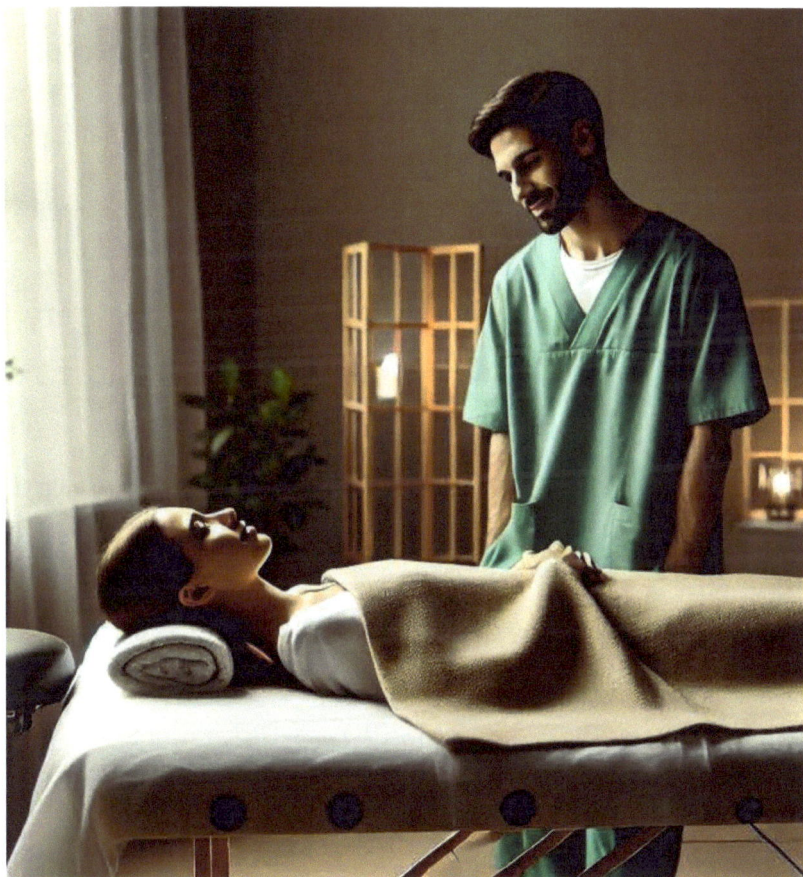

2. **Guidance from qualified professionals:** It is essential that manual lymphatic drainage be performed by a qualified and experienced professional. A massage therapist specializing in MLD understands the anatomy and specific needs of the lymphatic system and can apply the technique safely

and effectively. Additionally, the professional must be aware of the type of surgery performed and the particularities of the patient's case, ensuring that MLD is appropriate and beneficial.

3. **Considerations about the type of surgery:** The type of plastic surgery performed can influence both the timing and frequency of lymphatic drainage sessions. Let's explore some of the most common procedures and their recommendations:

- **Liposuction:** After liposuction, it is common for swelling to persist. MLD can be started generally between 48 to 72 hours after the procedure, with frequent sessions, usually recommended two to three times a week, depending on the level of swelling.

- **Abdominoplasty:** For abdominoplasties, drainage can be started in a similar period. As swelling tends to be more pronounced, regular sessions are recommended in the weeks following surgery.

- **Breast augmentation:** After the placement of breast implants, MLD can also be started around 48 to 72 hours after surgery. The focus should be on reducing swelling and improving healing, with regular sessions as needed.
- **Facelift:** For facial surgeries, drainage can begin a little earlier, around 48 hours after surgery, helping to minimize facial swelling and promote a better aesthetic appearance more quickly.

4. **Duration and Frequency of Sessions:** The duration and frequency of manual lymphatic drainage sessions can vary. In general, it is recommended:

- **Duration:** Each session can last between 30 to 60 minutes, depending on the area to be treated and the severity of the swelling.
- **Initial Frequency:** During the first week, sessions can be performed daily or on alternate days. After this period, the frequency can be adjusted to two to three times a week, depending on the patient's

recovery and the professional's recommendation.

5. **Signs of better recovery:** It is important that the patient be attentive to signs of improvement during the MLD process. The reduction of swelling, the decrease in pain, and the improvement in mobility are indicators that drainage is working. Additionally, the patient should report any discomfort or adverse reaction to the responsible professional, who can adjust the treatment as necessary.

6. **Contraindications and Precautions:** Although MLD is beneficial for many patients, there are some contraindications to consider. Patients with active infections, deep vein thrombosis, or certain medical conditions should avoid lymphatic drainage until a doctor authorizes it. Therefore, always consult the surgeon before starting MLD, ensuring that all health conditions are considered.

Conclusion

Manual lymphatic drainage is a valuable tool for post-operative recovery, and knowing when to start it can make all the difference in the healing process. With the guidance of qualified professionals and consideration of the type of surgery, patients can benefit greatly from this technique, accelerating their recovery and improving their aesthetic results. In the next chapter, we will address the specific indications and contraindications of manual lymphatic drainage, helping readers better understand when this technique is most appropriate.

Chapter 7

Contraindications and Necessary Precautions

Manual lymphatic drainage (MLD) is a generally safe and effective technique, especially in the context of post-operative recovery. However, like any treatment, there are contraindications and precautions that must be observed to ensure the safety and effectiveness of the procedure. In this chapter, we will address the main contraindications of MLD, the necessary precautions before starting treatment, and the importance of professional evaluation.

1. **General Contraindications:** It is crucial that manual lymphatic drainage be avoided in some specific situations. Among the main contraindications are:

    - **Active infectlons:** Patients with skin infections, systemic infections, or any active inflammatory condition should avoid MLD until the infection is treated and resolved.

Massage can spread the infection and worsen the condition.

- **Deep Vein Thrombosis (DVT):** MLD should not be applied to patients who have or have recently had deep vein thrombosis, as massage can destabilize the clot and increase the risk of serious complications.
- **Cancer:** Patients with active cancer should consult their doctor before starting MLD. Although lymphatic drainage can be beneficial in some situations, it should be performed with caution and only under medical supervision.
- **Heart Disease:** Severe heart conditions, such as congestive heart failure, may contraindicate MLD. Increased lymphatic flow can overload the cardiovascular system.
- **Hyperthermia:** If the patient is experiencing fever or any condition that causes an increase in body temperature, MLD should be avoided until the situation is stabilized.

2. Necessary Precautions: Before starting manual lymphatic drainage, it is essential that the massage therapist take some precautions and perform a complete assessment of the patient's health status.

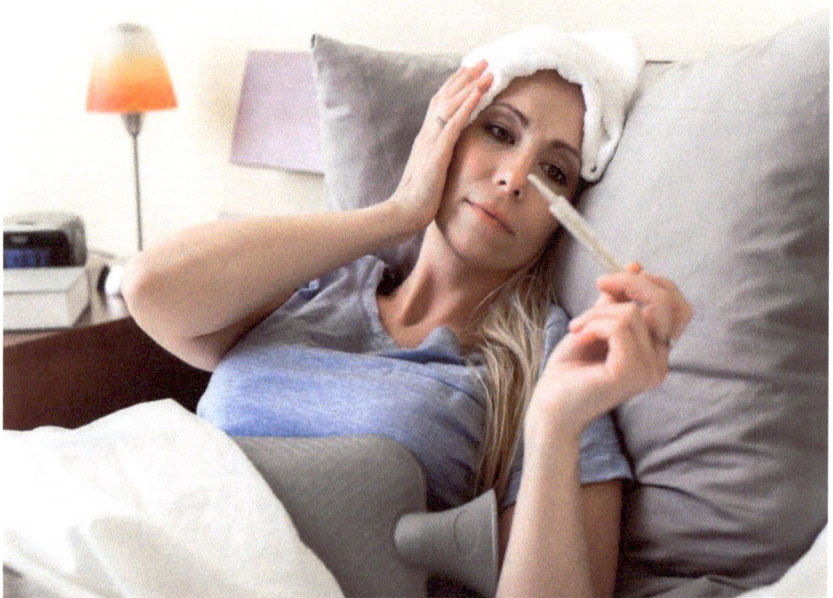

Here are some essential precautions:

- **Initial evaluation:** The massage therapist should conduct a detailed evaluation, including the patient's medical history, pre-existing conditions, medications in use, and the type of surgery performed, if applicable.
- **Medical consultation:** It is recommended that patients consult their surgeon or

responsible physician before starting MLD. This consultation is crucial to ensure that there are no contraindications and that the patient is fit to receive the treatment.

- **Open communication:** Patients should be encouraged to communicate any concerns or symptoms they are experiencing before and during MLD sessions. This includes intense pain, adverse reactions, or any change in health status.

3. **Precautions in Treatment:** During lymphatic drainage sessions, the massage therapist should follow some precautions to ensure patient safety:

- **Gentle movements:** MLD is characterized by light and rhythmic movements. Excessive pressure should be avoided, especially in areas where there is sensitivity or swelling.
- **Monitoring of reactions:** The professional should continuously monitor the patient's reaction during the session, adjusting the technique as necessary.

- **Adequate intervals:** It is important that sessions are scheduled so that the patient has enough time to recover between them. This helps to avoid overloading the lymphatic system.

4. **Importance of Professional Training:** The training and experience of the massage therapist are crucial to ensure patient safety. Qualified professionals should have a good understanding of contraindications and best practices in MLD. Continuous training and updating on new research and techniques are essential to ensure that patients receive the safest and most effective treatment possible.

Conclusion

Manual lymphatic drainage can be a powerful tool in post-operative recovery, but it is essential to approach treatment with caution. Knowing the contraindications and taking the necessary precautions are fundamental steps to ensure patient safety. With proper evaluation and monitoring by qualified professionals, MLD can offer significant benefits, contributing to a faster and more effective recovery. In the next chapter, we will discuss the specific techniques and approaches of manual lymphatic drainage, providing a deeper insight into how this practice is performed.

Chapter 8

The Manual Lymphatic Drainage Technique

Manual lymphatic drainage (MLD) is a therapeutic massage technique that aims to stimulate the lymphatic system, promoting the elimination of accumulated fluids and toxins from the body. This chapter will address the main movements used in MLD, the direction of flow, the intensity of maneuvers, and the importance of performing the technique gently and efficiently.

1. **Fundamental Principles of Lymphatic Drainage:** MLD is based on anatomical and physiological principles that guide the practice:

   - **Natural lymphatic flow:** The technique should always follow the direction of the natural flow of lymph, which moves towards the lymph nodes and, finally, back into the bloodstream.

- **Gentleness of movements:** The movements should be light and gentle, respecting the sensitivity of the lymphatic system and promoting a relaxing effect. Excessive pressure can cause discomfort and even impair lymphatic flow.

2. **Main Movements of Lymphatic Drainage:** There are several characteristic movements of MLD, each with a specific purpose:

- **Static pressure:** This movement consists of applying light pressure to the skin, usually in areas with a higher concentration of lymph nodes. The goal is to prepare the area for drainage and stimulate lymph circulation. The pressure should be constant and gentle, lasting a few seconds.
- **Pumping movements:** Pumping movements are used to stimulate lymphatic flow towards the nodes. They involve a sequence of rhythmic pressures, where the hands move down and up in a smooth pattern. These movements are especially effective in extremities such as arms and legs.

- **Gliding:** Gliding movements are continuous and smooth movements that follow the direction of lymphatic flow. The palms of the hands glide over the skin, applying light pressure. This movement is ideal for larger areas, such as the abdomen and back, and helps to facilitate fluid drainage.

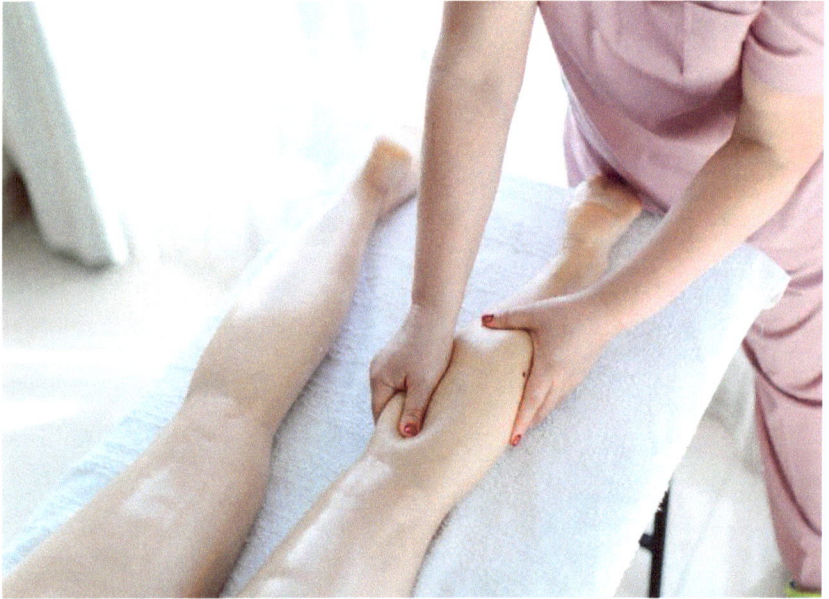

- **Gentle twists:** Gentle twists involve rotational movements on extremities, such as arms and legs. These movements help release tension in muscles and stimulate lymphatic drainage, being effective for areas where fluid can accumulate.

47

- **Landing and return:** This movement is characterized by a light touch and a gentle removal of the hands, allowing the skin to relax between maneuvers. It can be used to finish a session, providing a feeling of comfort and well-being.

3. **Direction of Flow:** In manual lymphatic drainage, the direction of flow is fundamental. Lymph flows from peripheral areas towards the heart and lymph nodes. Therefore, movements should always be directed:

- **From extremities to the center:** When working on arms and legs, the movements should go towards the armpit or groin, where the lymph nodes are located.

- **From top to bottom:** In the abdomen and back, the movements should be performed in a way that helps the flow of lymph towards the lymph nodes of the thoracic region.

- **Intensity of maneuvers:** The intensity of maneuvers should be adjusted according to the patient's sensitivity. The general rule is that pressure should be light. The main points to consider include:

- **Patient comfort:** The massage therapist should always assess the patient's response during MLD. If there is discomfort, the pressure should be reduced.

- **Sensitive areas:** Some areas of the body may be more sensitive than others, especially after surgeries. It is crucial to adapt the intensity as needed.

4. **Importance of Professional Training:** The correct application of the manual lymphatic drainage technique requires proper training and practice.

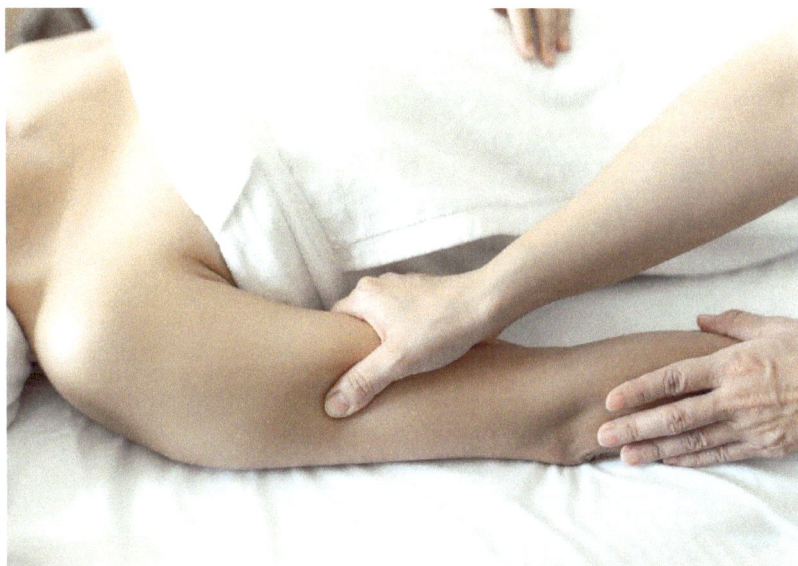

A qualified massage therapist must understand the anatomy of the lymphatic system and the best practices to apply MLD effectively and safely. Furthermore, adapting the technique to the patient's health status and individual needs is essential to optimize results.

Conclusion

Manual lymphatic drainage is a delicate technique that requires knowledge and skill. The combination of gentle movements, correct direction of flow, and adaptation of intensity are essential to ensure that

MLD offers all its benefits. By mastering these principles, the massage therapist can provide effective treatment, promoting recovery and well-being for patients.

In the next chapter, we will discuss the specific indications for MLD, detailing the conditions and situations in which this technique can be especially beneficial.

Chapter 9

Preparation for a Lymphatic Drainage Session

Proper preparation for a manual lymphatic drainage (MLD) session is essential to ensure that the treatment is effective and that the patient feels comfortable and safe. In this chapter, we will discuss the essential elements of preparation, including the choice of environment, the importance of hydration, and clear communication between the massage therapist and the patient.

1. **Choice of environment:** A suitable environment can make a big difference in the patient's experience during MLD. Here are some points to consider:

   - **Calm and cozy environment:** The place should be quiet, free from distractions and excessive noise. Soft lighting and a pleasant temperature help create a relaxing environment.

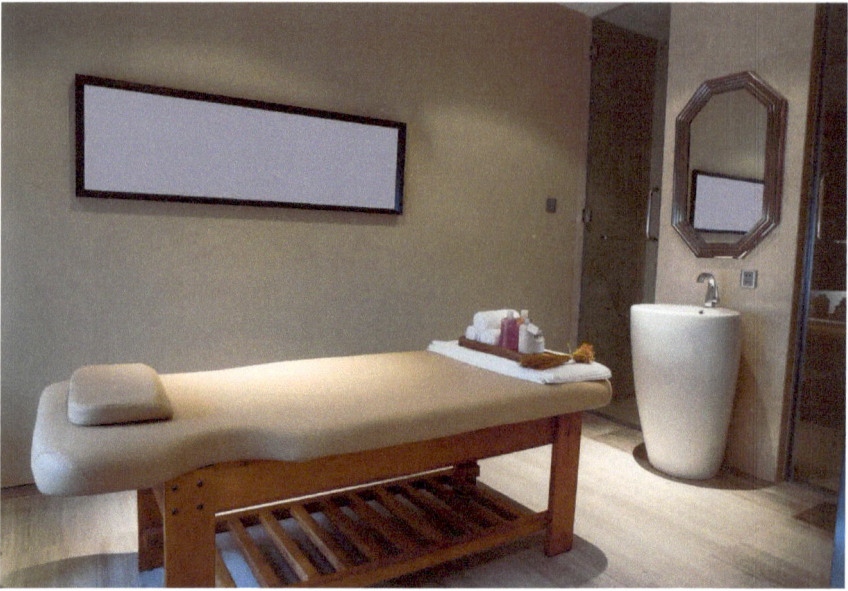

- **Cleanliness and comfort:** The room should be clean and organized, with a comfortable and suitable massage table. Clean and soft towels, as well as blankets, should be available to ensure patient comfort during the session.

- **Aromatherapy and soft music:** Some practices include the use of essential oils or soft music to promote relaxation. This can help create a welcoming and soothing atmosphere.

2. **Patient Hydration:** Hydration is a crucial aspect before a manual lymphatic drainage session. Here are some recommendations:

- **Water intake:** It is important that the patient is well hydrated before the session. Water helps to fluidize the lymph, facilitating its movement through the lymphatic system. It is recommended that the patient drink water in the hours leading up to the session.
- **Avoid dehydrating beverages:** Alcoholic and caffeinated beverages should be avoided, as they can cause dehydration, which can decrease the effectiveness of MLD.

3. **Clear Communication:** Effective communication between the massage therapist and the patient is essential to ensure that the MLD session meets the patient's needs and expectations. Some tips include:

- **Health history:** The massage therapist should ask questions about the patient's health history, including any medical conditions, recent surgeries, and medications in use. This will help to adapt the session to the patient's specific needs.
- **Session expectations:** The patient should be informed about what to expect during MLD. This includes the types of movements that will be performed, the duration of the session, and how they may feel during and after the treatment.
- **Feedback during the session:** The massage therapist should encourage the patient to provide feedback on the intensity and sensation of the movements. This continuous communication will help to adjust the technique as needed to maximize comfort and effectiveness.

4. **Clothing and Physical Preparation:** The way the patient dresses for the session can also impact the effectiveness of lymphatic drainage. Some guidelines include:

- **Comfortable clothing:** It is recommended that the patient wear loose and comfortable clothing that allows easy access to the areas to be treated, such as arms, legs, and abdomen.

- **Removal of accessories:** The patient should be instructed to remove jewelry and accessories that may interfere with the massage or cause discomfort.

5. **Mental Preparation:** Mental preparation is also an important component of the session. Some strategies that can help include:

- **Relaxation:** Relaxation techniques, such as deep breathing or meditation, can be recommended before the session to help the patient calm down and prepare for MLD.

- **Positive expectations:** The patient should be encouraged to maintain a positive mindset regarding the session and the expected results, which can influence the overall experience.

Conclusion

Preparation for a manual lymphatic drainage session is a key factor in ensuring the best possible results. A suitable environment, patient hydration, clear communication, and physical and mental comfort are all elements that contribute to a successful MLD experience. By preparing properly, both the massage therapist and the patient can work together to maximize the benefits of the technique. In the next chapter, we will discuss the specific indications of manual lymphatic drainage, exploring the conditions in which this technique can be especially beneficial.

Chaper 10

The Role of the Health Professional

Manual lymphatic drainage (MLD) is a powerful technique that can offer significant benefits in recovery and health promotion. However, the effectiveness of this treatment depends heavily on the competence and experience of the professional who performs it. In this chapter, we will discuss the importance of choosing a qualified massage therapist, with their proper licenses, and the impact that this choice can have on the safety and results of the treatment.

The Importance of Qualification

Training and specialization are fundamental aspects to consider when choosing a manual lymphatic drainage professional. A qualified massage therapist should have:

- **Formal education:** Training in massage therapy, with an emphasis on lymphatic drainage techniques. Recognized courses ensure that the professional understands the anatomy, physiology, and specific techniques necessary for MLD.

- **Certifications and licenses:** Relevant certifications and licenses that attest to the massage therapist's qualification are essential. This ensures that the professional is in compliance with local regulations and has received adequate training.
- **Experience and practice:** Practical experience is one of the main factors that contribute to the effectiveness of manual lymphatic drainage. Experienced massage therapists offer a range of benefits and in-depth knowledge. Professionals with years of experience have a deeper understanding of patients' challenges and needs, allowing them to adapt the MLD technique to specific situations.
- **Effective evaluation:** Experience allows the massage therapist to perform an accurate assessment of the patient's health status, identifying contraindications and adjusting the treatment as necessary.

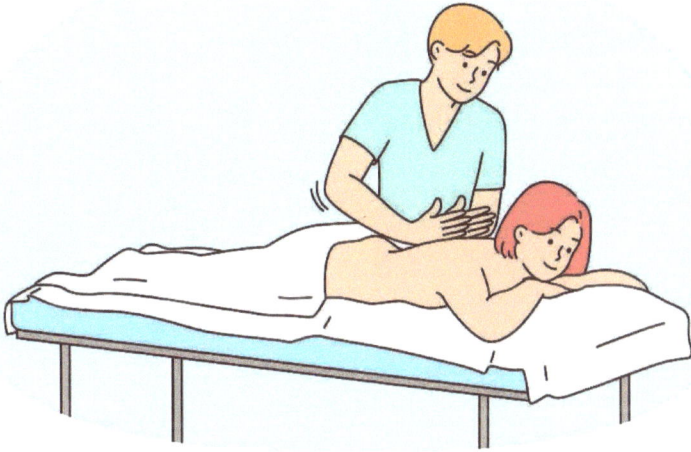

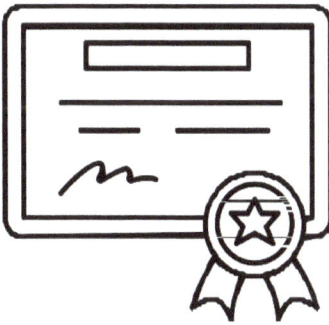

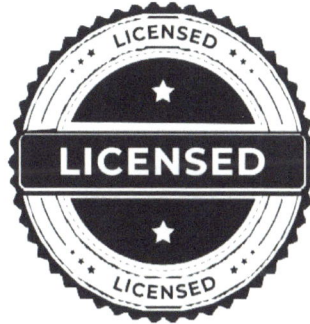

- **Consistent results:** Continued practice helps refine the massage therapist's skills, resulting in more effective treatments and better outcomes for patients.

Personalized Approach

Each patient is unique, and a qualified professional should be able to offer a personalized approach. This includes:

- **Complete anamnesis:** Conducting a detailed patient history to understand their specific needs, including recent surgeries, medical conditions, and expectations regarding treatment.

- **Adaptation of the technique:** An experienced massage therapist will adjust the MLD technique based on the patient's individual characteristics, such as sensitivity, areas of swelling, and pre-existing health conditions.

- **Education and guidance:** A good health professional not only performs the treatment but also educates the patient about the process, which includes:
  - **Explanation of the technique:** Informing the patient about the movements that will be performed, the importance of lymphatic drainage, and

what they can expect during and after the session.

- ○ **Post-treatment care:** Providing guidance on care to be followed after MLD, such as the importance of hydration, light exercise, and other practices that can optimize results.

Trust and Safety

The relationship of trust between the patient and the massage therapist is fundamental. Patients who feel safe and comfortable are more likely to relax and achieve better results. A reputable professional should:

- **Promote a safe environment:** Create a space where the patient feels comfortable expressing their concerns and asking questions about the treatment.
- **Respect professional ethics:** Maintain high standards of ethics, confidentiality, and respect for the patient's needs and limits.

Conclusion

Choosing a qualified professional for manual lymphatic drainage is a fundamental step to ensure safe and effective treatment. Experience, knowledge, and the ability to personalize care are essential characteristics that contribute to maximizing the benefits of MLD.

Experienced and well-trained professionals are examples of how to achieve positive results, helping patients on their journey of recovery and well-being. In the end, collaboration between the patient and the massage therapist is the key to a successful treatment experience, promoting health and vitality.

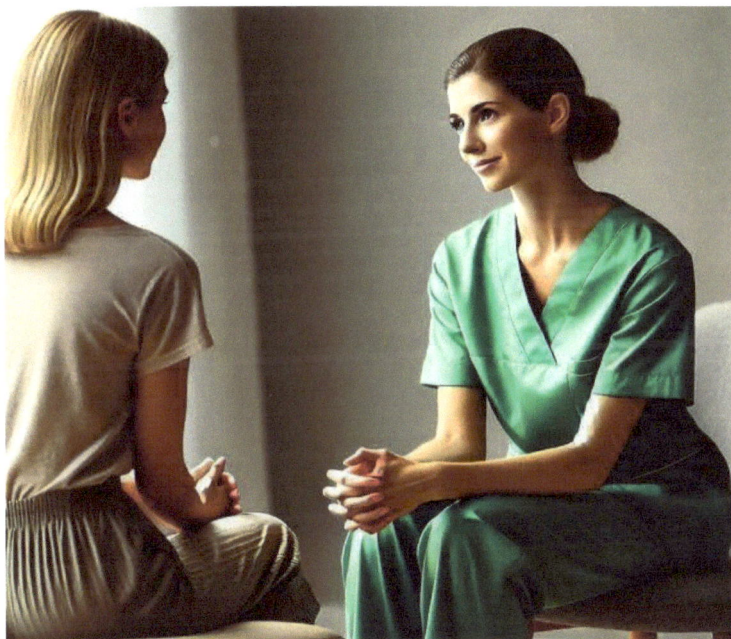

Chapter 11

Patient Experiences

Testimonials

"Lymphatic drainage therapy was transformative for my knees. I was skeptical. After several knee surgeries and procedures, I was told to have a knee replacement. After 5 sessions, I am walking without pain, my range of motion has increased to almost 100%, and I am now active again."
Edgard Ochoa

"Mario does an incredible job as a therapist; I have been his patient since 2012 (...) in our sessions, he has done an excellent job, in which I was able to walk without limping and without pain. Thanks to Mario's lymphatic massages, I have started living a normal life, without painkillers and surgeries." **Vickie Santos**

" Very professional and effective lymphatic massage. Definitely recommend!" **Jacque Alvarez**

"Thank you so much, Mario, for my first real lymphatic massage!!! After my 360-liposuction surgery, I had 15 massages with someone else and was still big and swollen. Then I looked for Mario after hearing such good things about him... After a real lymphatic drainage massage from Mario, I feel better than the 15 bad massages from someone else made me feel... Thank you so much, Mario, see you next week... And thank you for all the knowledge you passed on to me about the human body." **Nicole Stewart**

"Mario is very talented at what he does. He helped me through a very difficult health time in 2017/2018. I really appreciate his dedication to healing and can't wait to go back for more lymphatic treatments." **Dee Pittman**

"Absolutely amazing! You leave feeling totally new!" **Aurejana Ceaser**

"Mario is an accomplished professional and a talented lymphatic masseur. If I could give more than 5 stars, I would! If you are investing in surgery, you MUST use him before and after the procedure. I am having wonderful results and am on day 28 post-procedure, and this would not have been possible without Mario. I cannot recommend him enough!" **Catherine Lenihan**

"Mario is great! I had a lymphatic massage a few days after rotator cuff surgery. After just one session, I was able to close my hand completely after, whereas before I could barely move my swollen fingers. Two more sessions eliminated the swelling in my arm. My physical therapist was impressed. He's a nice guy too." **Victor H.**

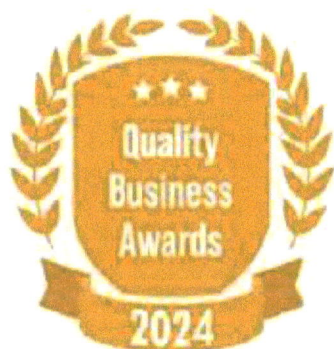

Quality Business Awards 2024

LYMPHATIC MASSAGE CENTER

Kenner

3712 Williams Blvd Ste H, Kenner, LA 70065

We have awarded Lymphatic Massage Center as The Best Massage Therapist in Kenner for 2024. An overall quality score exceeding 95% was achieved, making them the top ranked in Kenner

★★★★★ **Satisfaction**

★★★★★ **Service**

★★★★★ **Reputation**

★★★★★ **Quality**

Chapter 12

Lymphatic Drainage and Aesthetics:

A Holistic Approach:

Manual lymphatic drainage (MLD) is not just an isolated technique, but a practice that can be integrated with a variety of aesthetic and therapeutic approaches, promoting a holistic view of health and well-being. In this chapter, we will explore how MLD complements other aesthetic practices, the benefits of this integration, and how a holistic approach can improve patients' quality of life.

1. The Interconnection Between Lymphatic Drainage and Aesthetics

A Manual lymphatic drainage plays a significant role in aesthetics, especially in treatments aimed at beauty and skin health. The technique not only helps reduce swelling and improve circulation but can also enhance the results of other aesthetic treatments:

- **Improved skin appearance:** MLD promotes the elimination of toxins and accumulated fluids, which can result in healthier, more radiant skin. By stimulating the lymphatic system, MLD can improve skin texture and tone, contributing to an overall more rejuvenated appearance.
- **Integration with aesthetic treatments:** MLD can be performed before or after aesthetic procedures, such as fillers, Botox, or laser treatments, to optimize results. Drainage can help reduce swelling and sensitivity after these procedures, accelerating recovery and improving aesthetic outcomes.

2. Combination with Wellness Practices

MLD can be combined with other wellness practices to promote a state of physical and emotional balance. Some of these practices include:

- **Relaxing massages:** Integrating MLD with relaxing or therapeutic massages can provide a more complete relaxation experience. This combination helps relieve stress and muscle tension, creating an environment conducive to recovery.
- **Aromatherapy:** The use of essential oils during MLD can amplify the benefits of the technique. Aromatherapy not only promotes relaxation but can also have properties that aid in detoxification and stress relief, enhancing the effects of lymphatic drainage.
- **Holistic therapies:** MLD can be part of a broader regimen that includes practices such as yoga, Pilates, or meditation. These practices, when combined, promote harmony between body and mind, helping to maintain a healthy and balanced lifestyle.

3. Healthy Lifestyle

Integrating manual lymphatic drainage into a holistic aesthetic approach also involves adopting a healthy lifestyle. Some recommendations include:

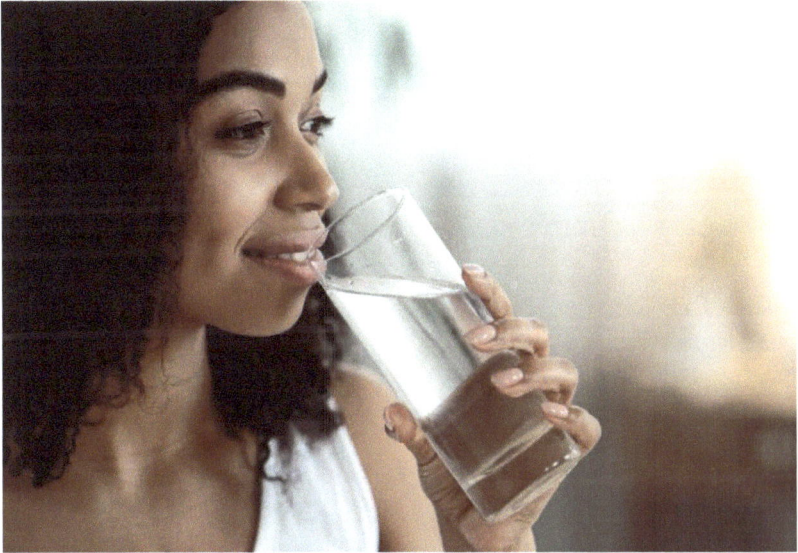

- **Proper hydration:** Water intake is crucial to optimize the benefits of MLD. Hydration helps keep the lymphatic system functioning properly, facilitating the elimination of toxins and promoting healthy skin.

- **Balanced diet:** A diet rich in fruits, vegetables, and anti-inflammatory foods can help the lymphatic system. Foods like avocado, nuts, and omega-3-rich fish are beneficial for overall health and can complement the effects of lymphatic drainage.

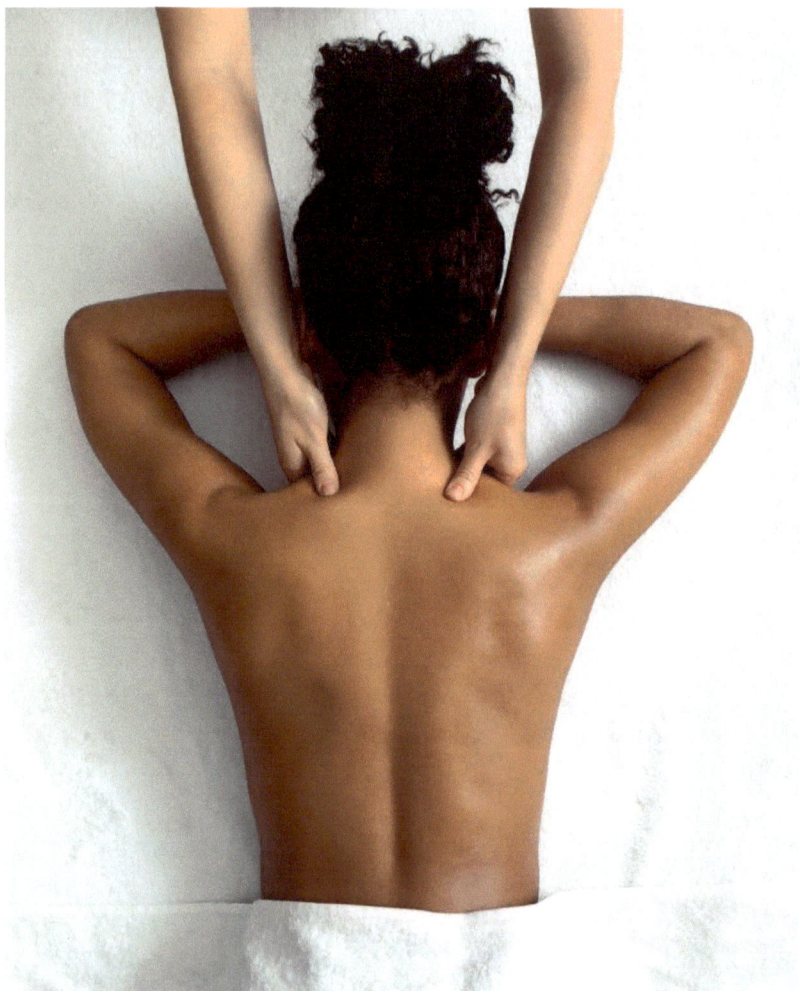

●

- **Regular exercise:** Physical activity is essential to stimulate the lymphatic system. Regular exercise helps promote circulation and the elimination of toxins, enhancing the results of MLD.

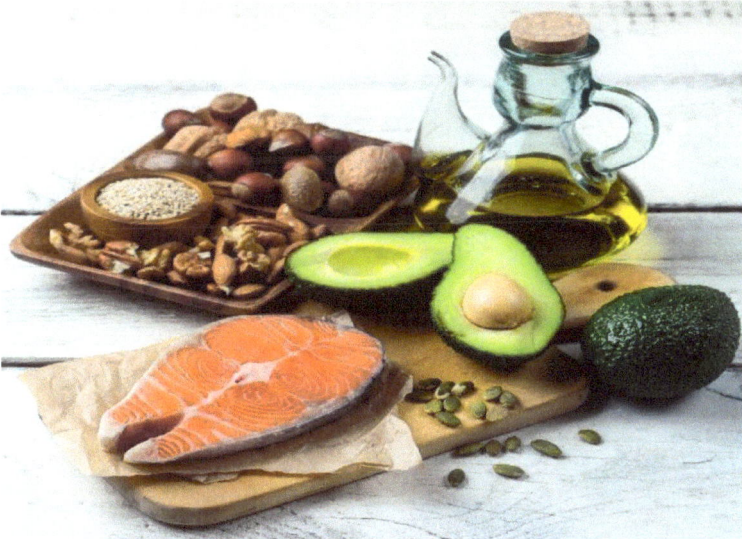

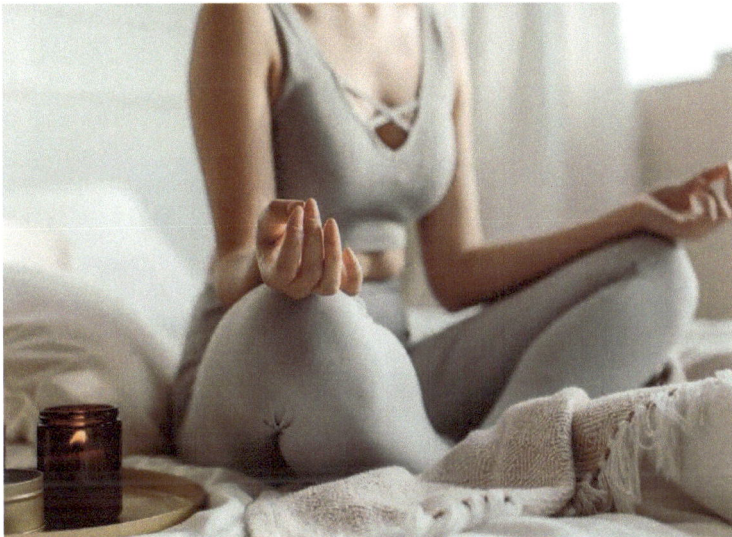

4. Emotional Benefits

A holistic approach to lymphatic drainage also recognizes the emotional benefits that the technique can offer. The deep relaxation promoted by MLD can help reduce anxiety and stress, leading to improved mental health. Patients frequently report feeling more balanced and rejuvenated after sessions.

5. Final Considerations

Manual lymphatic drainage can be a central element in a holistic aesthetic approach, offering benefits that go beyond physical appearance.

By integrating MLD with other aesthetic and wellness practices, patients can experience a transformation that encompasses not only the body but also the mind and spirit. This integrated approach not only promotes health and beauty but also encourages a balanced and sustainable lifestyle. As we conclude this chapter, it is clear that manual lymphatic drainage is not just a massage technique; it is an essential part of a broader path to well-being and aesthetics.

In the next chapter, we will reflect on the evolution of lymphatic drainage and its future perspectives in the field of health and aesthetics.

Chapter 13

Common Questions About Lymphatic Drainage

Manual lymphatic drainage (MLD) is a technique that, despite its widely recognized benefits, still generates many doubts and misinformation. In this chapter, we will address some of the most frequently asked questions about MLD, demystifying myths and clarifying important points so that you can better understand this practice and its effects.

1. What is Manual Lymphatic Drainage?

Question: What exactly is manual lymphatic drainage?

Answer: Manual lymphatic drainage is a gentle massage technique that aims to stimulate the flow of lymph, a fluid that carries toxins and waste from the body. The technique uses rhythmic and gentle movements, directed at the lymphatic vessels, helping to eliminate excess fluids and improve circulation.

2. What are the benefits of lymphatic drainage?

Question: What are the main benefits of lymphatic drainage?

Answer: The benefits include reducing swelling, improving blood circulation, relieving pain, accelerating post-surgical recovery, and promoting deep relaxation. MLD can also help improve skin appearance, contributing to a healthier look.

3. Is Lymphatic Drainage only for those who have had plastic surgery?

Question: Is lymphatic drainage only indicated for people who have undergone plastic surgery?

Answer: No. Although MLD is highly recommended in the post-operative period to aid in recovery, it can be beneficial for anyone who experiences swelling, fluid retention, or imbalances in the lymphatic system. The technique is also used in cases of cellulite, edema, and for general aesthetic purposes.

4. Is it a painful technique?

Question: Is manual lymphatic drainage painful?

Answer: No. MLD is a gentle and painless technique. The movements are performed delicately, and most patients report feelings of relaxation and relief during and after the session. If the technique causes discomfort, it is important to communicate with the professional for adjustments in intensity.

5. How many sessions are necessary?

Question: How many lymphatic drainage sessions are recommended?

Answer: The number of sessions can vary depending on individual needs and the type of treatment desired. For post-surgical patients, several sessions may be recommended in a short period, while for maintenance and well-being, one to two sessions per month may be sufficient.

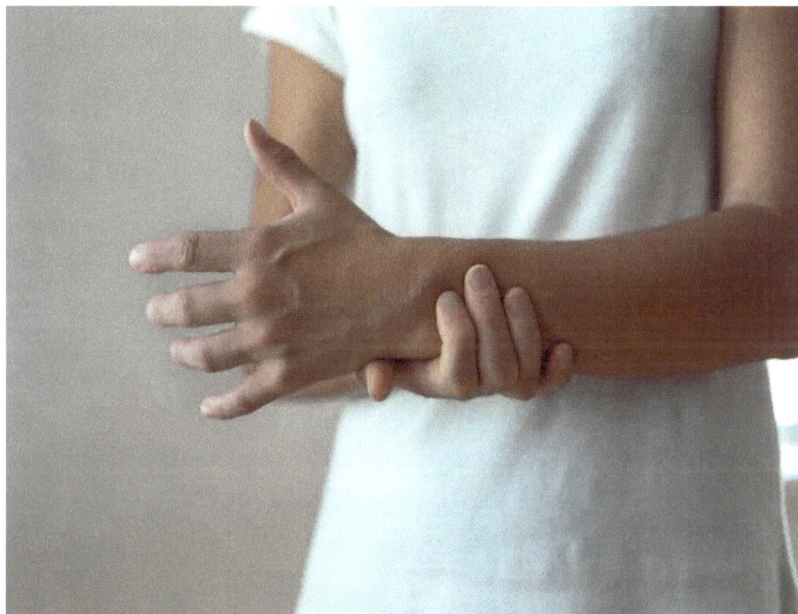

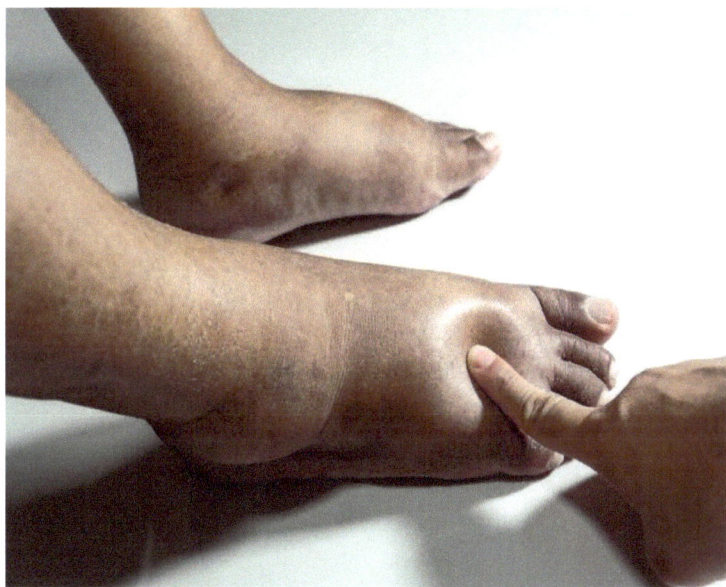

6. Are there contraindications for Lymphatic Drainage?

Question: Are there contraindications for lymphatic drainage?

Answer: Yes. While MLD is safe for many people, there are contraindications, such as infections, heart problems, deep vein thrombosis, and some autoimmune conditions. It is essential that the massage therapist perform a complete evaluation before starting treatment.

7. Can I do lymphatic drainage at home?

Question: Is it possible to perform lymphatic drainage at home?

Answer: Although there are lymphatic drainage techniques that can be done at home, such as self-massages, it is always recommended to seek a qualified professional, especially after surgery or for specific conditions. The massage therapist has the knowledge necessary to apply the technique effectively and safely.

8. Does lymphatic drainage help you lose weight?

Question: Can lymphatic drainage help with weight loss?

Answer: MLD is not a weight loss technique, but it can help reduce fluid retention and swelling, creating a more sculpted appearance. For effective weight loss, it is important to combine MLD with a healthy diet and regular exercise.

9. Can I do lymphatic drainage during menstruation?

Question: Can lymphatic drainage be done during the menstrual period?

Answer: Yes, but this can vary from person to person. Some women may feel more sensitive during menstruation and prefer to avoid sessions. It is important to communicate your preferences to the massage therapist.

10. How to choose a good professional?

Question: How can I choose a good massage therapist for lymphatic drainage?

Answer: Look for a qualified professional, with specific training in lymphatic drainage and experience in post-surgical or aesthetic treatments. Also, check references and testimonials from other patients to ensure you are choosing someone reliable.

Conclusion

Doubts and myths surrounding manual lymphatic drainage are common, but it is important to seek accurate information to better understand this technique and its benefits. By clarifying these issues, we hope that you feel more confident and prepared to consider MLD as part of your health and wellness journey.

In the next chapter, we will address the future perspectives of lymphatic drainage and its evolution in the field of health and aesthetics.

Chapter 14

The Future of Manual Lymphatic Drainage

Manual lymphatic drainage (MLD) is a practice that has solidified over the years, but its evolution is far from stagnant. With the advancement of research and therapeutic techniques, the future of MLD promises innovations that will not only enhance the effectiveness of the treatment but also expand its applications and benefits. In this chapter, we will explore emerging trends, new techniques, and the integration of MLD with other treatment modalities.

1. Advances in research

Research in manual lymphatic drainage is intensifying, with studies seeking to better understand the physiological mechanisms behind the technique. This includes investigations into how MLD affects the immune system, wound healing, and the management of chronic conditions.

As more data is collected, it will be possible to develop evidence-based protocols that will ensure more effective treatment.

2. Emerging Technologies

Technology is playing an increasing role in the evolution of lymphatic drainage. The use of electronic devices to simulate the manual movements of MLD is already in use in several clinics and spas. These devices, such as pneumatic compression devices, can provide effective and accessible treatment, especially for those who do not have access to qualified professionals.

3. Integration with other therapies

MLD is increasingly integrating with other therapeutic modalities, creating a multidisciplinary approach to well-being. For example:

- **Aesthetic therapies:** MLD can be combined with treatments such as radiofrequency, ultrasound, and laser therapy, enhancing results and improving recovery.
- **Holistic therapies**: The integration of MLD with practices such as acupuncture, aromatherapy, and yoga can offer a more

complete care experience, promoting physical and emotional balance.

4. Education and Professional Training

The future of MLD also involves a greater emphasis on education and professional training. As the technique becomes more popular, the need for well-trained and qualified massage therapists increases. Training and certification programs are expanding, ensuring that professionals have a solid knowledge of anatomy, physiology, and MLD techniques.

5. Expansion of Clinical Applications

In addition to its aesthetic applications, MLD is being recognized as a valuable therapy in various clinical areas. Recent research suggests that MLD may be beneficial in cases of lymphedema, arthritis, fibromyalgia, and other conditions involving inflammation and fluid retention. The expansion of clinical indications can lead to greater recognition of MLD as an essential therapeutic practice in integrative medicine.

6. Personalização do Tratamento

As knowledge about lymphatic drainage advances, it is expected that treatment will become increasingly personalized. Detailed patient assessments, including lifestyle analysis, pre-existing health conditions, and specific goals, will allow massage therapists to adjust MLD sessions to better meet individual needs.

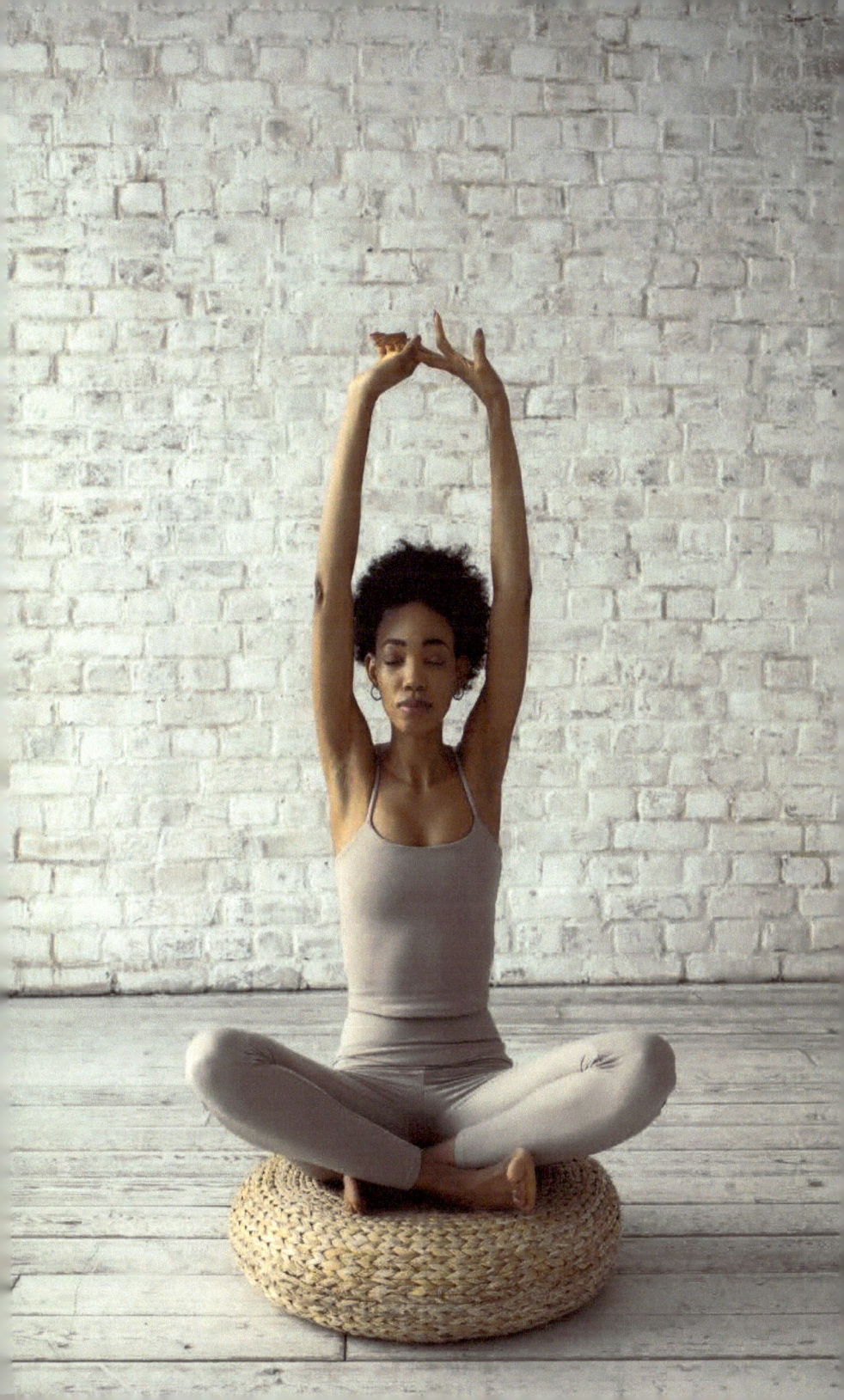

7. Awareness and Access: With the growing awareness of the benefits of manual lymphatic drainage, it is expected that there will be an expansion of access to this therapy.

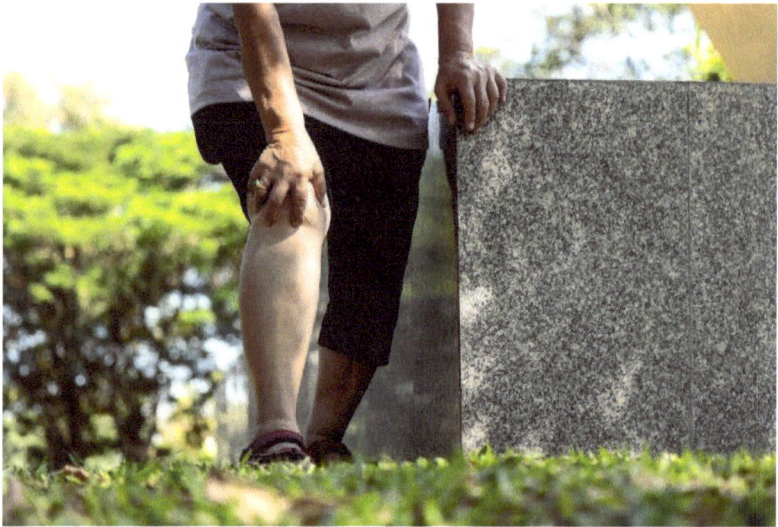

Public awareness programs and community health initiatives can help educate people about the importance of MLD, especially for those recovering from surgery or dealing with chronic conditions.

Conclusion

The future of manual lymphatic drainage is promising, with innovations and advances that expand its applications and increase its effectiveness. As more people seek treatments that promote health and well-being, MLD will consolidate as a valuable and accessible therapeutic option.

With the continuous evolution of techniques and the strengthening of professional training, manual lymphatic drainage will be able to reach new levels, benefiting more and more patients in their journeys of recovery and self-care. In the next and final chapter, we will reflect on the importance of manual lymphatic drainage in health and well-being, consolidating everything we have learned throughout this book.

Chapter 15

Conclusion: The Importance of Proper Recovery

As we reach the end of this book, it is essential to reflect on the importance of proper recovery, especially after plastic surgeries and aesthetic procedures. Manual lymphatic drainage (MLD) stands out as an essential tool in this process, contributing to the physical and emotional well-being of patients.

The Need for Post-Surgical Care

Recovery after plastic surgery is not limited to the time the body takes to heal. It involves a series of care measures that ensure not only physical recovery but also the restoration of emotional balance. In this context, MLD emerges as a valuable intervention, helping to reduce swelling, improve circulation, and accelerate the healing process.

Proven Benefits of Lymphatic Drainage

As discussed throughout the chapters, the benefits of MLD go beyond aesthetics. This technique:

- **Promotes the elimination of toxins:** helps in the removal of waste and toxins accumulated in the body, allowing for a healthier recovery.
- **Reduces edema and swelling:** MLD decreases fluid retention, providing relief and comfort.
- **Accelerates healing:** stimulates blood circulation, promoting tissue oxygenation and accelerating cell regeneration.
- **Offers emotional relief:** the gentle touch of drainage not only relaxes the body but also calms the mind, helping to reduce anxiety and stress.

The Importance of Professional Choice

A crucial point we emphasized throughout the book is the importance of choosing a qualified professional to perform lymphatic drainage. The experience and knowledge of a trained massage therapist ensure that the treatment is safe and effective, maximizing the benefits for the patient. Trust in the professional is fundamental for the recovery experience to be positive and productive.

Integration of Practices

Another important aspect is the integration of MLD with other health and aesthetic practices. By combining lymphatic drainage with physical exercises, healthy eating, and other therapies, patients can achieve a more complete state of well-being. The holistic approach, which considers the body and mind, is proving increasingly effective in promoting health.

Looking to the Future

As MLD continues to evolve, new techniques and research will expand its applications and benefits. The future promises not only improvements in lymphatic drainage practices but also a growing recognition of its importance in integrative medicine and aesthetics. With this, more and more people will be able to benefit from the positive effects of MLD in their lives.

Final Reflection

In summary, manual lymphatic drainage proves to be a powerful ally in recovery and self-care. By addressing health holistically, recognizing the interconnection between body and mind, we can provide patients with a more complete and satisfying recovery experience. By investing in proper recovery, patients not only heal physically but also promote a healthier and more balanced lifestyle. The recovery journey is unique for each individual, but with the right tools and adequate support, it is possible to transform this process into an opportunity for growth and renewal.

May this book serve as a guide for all who seek to better understand manual lymphatic drainage and its significant contributions to health and well-being.

Book Conclusion

In this book, we explored manual lymphatic drainage (MLD) in depth, from its fundamentals and benefits to its specific importance in post-operative plastic surgery.

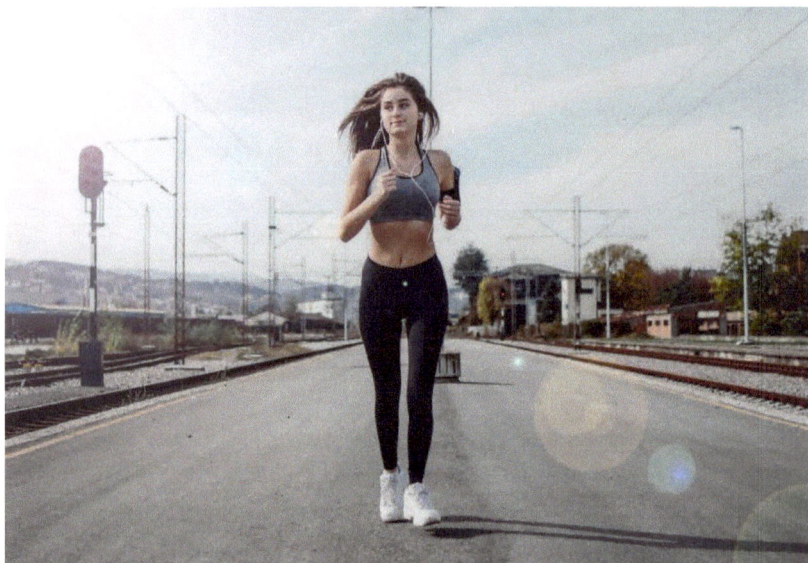

Throughout the chapters, we discussed the anatomy of the lymphatic system, the drainage technique, its contraindications and necessary care, and even the experiences of patients who experienced the positive effects of this practice. MLD is not just an aesthetic technique; it is an integral approach that promotes health and well-being. Its benefits go beyond reducing swelling and improving healing; it contributes to a state of relaxation and emotional balance. With the increased recognition of MLD as a valuable tool in recovery, choosing a qualified professional becomes essential to ensure effective and safe results.

As we look to the future, it is evident that manual lymphatic drainage is constantly evolving, keeping pace with new research and technological innovations. This growth will not only expand its applications but also make MLD an increasingly accessible practice for everyone.

We hope that this book has provided a clear and comprehensive understanding of manual lymphatic drainage, encouraging self-care and the pursuit of a more balanced state of health. By investing in proper recovery, each individual can transform their healing process into an opportunity for renewal and well-being. May MLD be a step towards a healthier and fuller life.